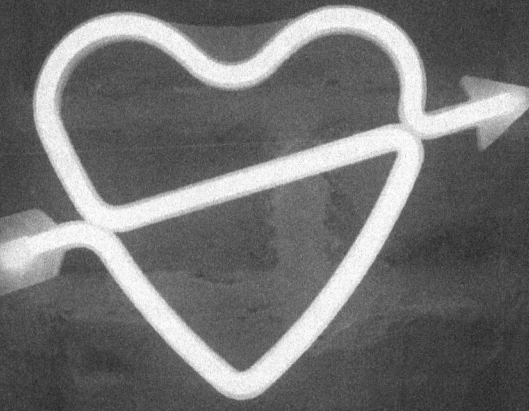

Twin Horseshoes Publishing
www.twinhorseshoes.ca
Ontario, Canada

Copyright © Listen to Your F*CKing HEART, 2025

All rights reserved. Without limiting the rights under copyright reserved above, no part of this publication may be reproduced, stored in, or introduced into a retrieval system, or transmitted in any form or by any means (electronic, mechanical, including photocopying, recording or otherwise), without the prior written permission of both the copyright owner and the above publisher of this book.

This publication contains the opinions and ideas of its author and is designed to provide useful information in regard to the subject matter covered. The author and publisher are not engaged in professional services in this publication. This publication is not intended to provide a basis for action in particular circumstances without consideration by a competent professional. The author and publisher expressly disclaim any responsibility for any liability, loss, or risk, personal or otherwise, which is incurred as a consequence, directly or indirectly, of the use and application of any of the contents of this book. While the author has made every effort to provide accurate information at publication time, the publisher and the author assume no responsibility for third-party websites or their content.

Nancy Seibel
Listen to Your F*CKing HEART:
Finding Yourself, Growing Daily, & Making the Choice to Love

Includes bibliographical references.

eBook ISBN 978-1-990831-08-9
Paperback ISBN 978-1-7778033-1-5

Health, Fitness & Dieting › Alternative Medicine › Healing
Parenting & Relationships › Parenting › Emotions & Feelings
Self-Help › Personal Transformation

chronic pain, trauma, epigenetics, authenticity, misalignment, mindfulness, resilience

This book is sold subject to the condition that it shall not, by way of trade or otherwise, be lent, re-sold, hired out, or otherwise circulated without the publisher's prior consent in any form of binding or cover other than that in which it is published and without a similar condition including this condition being imposed on the subsequent purchase.

Dedication

To the AMAZING, INCREDIBLE, STRONG WARRIORS who are my daughters, you are my everything and it's been my mission from the day I was born to be the best MOMMA for my girls. I think I've become the best MOMMA because of the amazing lessons I've learned from the 2 of you...I've made mistakes, I've grown, I've learned, but one thing is for certain—I couldn't have done it without you and your love and support. We are so blessed to have what we have, Winston and Harley included. I love our ability to have the best conversations, and we can talk about pretty much anything...but more importantly, I love how much we respect one another. Thank you for teaching me how important it is to be authentic in everything I do and thank you for reminding me what unconditional love is supposed to FEEL like. This journey has not been easy and the whirlwind roller coaster of life we've lived has taught us all a lot and yet, my only hope now is for PEACE, LOVE, JOY, and for our DREAMS coming true. I love you. I am proud of you. Know that all I want for you both is to be your best and most authentic selves.

Know that I'm always here for you both…I never want US to change—unconditional love forever and always…

To my Mom, unconditional love is our superpower and what a journey we've had together. I couldn't do this without you. I wouldn't be here without you, and I'm grateful for everything you've done for me to become ME again. You've never stopped being my guide in the darkness and, more importantly, you've believed in me even when I couldn't believe in myself. You've truly taught me all the powerful lessons that have wound up in this book—I've just taken them and shaken them up…Nancy style. Thank you for your love and for your commitment to being the best mom. Both Jenny and I truly are blessed for your love and support.

Thank you to everyone who has been on my journey—even those whose chapters with me didn't end well. I am blessed for your love and more importantly your lessons as they've made me ME and being ME has become my greatest superpower. I hope that if we see each other after you read this, we flow with even more HEART together and realize how important love is vs. anything else. The time really is NOW.

Contents

Introduction 9
PART 1: HUMAN 17
  Chapter 1: The Universe Keeps Knocking 19
    We Can Only Go So Far 21
    THERE IS NO YOU, WITHOUT YOU 23
    …Until You Listen 25
      HEART: 180 Degrees... 26
  Chapter 2: What is Your Body Trying to Tell You?..... 27
    From Numb, to Pain, and Beyond 29
    Misalignment... 32
    Empower Yourself.. 35
      HEART: Listen to Your Body.............................. 37
PART 2: EMPOWERMENT 39
  Chapter 3: My Unravelling.. 41
    Superwoman 42
    Great "Mom" Expectations 45
    A Dose of Reality 48
      HEART: Superpower Playlist 52
      HEART: Great Expectations................................ 53
  Chapter 4: Do it For You AND Your Family................ 55
    The Mirror... 57
    Epigenetics... 58
    Go Inward... 60

  HEART: Look in the Mirror 63
  HEART: Tune In 64
PART 3: ALIGNMENT 65
 Chapter 5: The BIG Job 67
  The Dream 68
  Set Up to Fail 69
  Authentic Self 73
  HEART: Re-alignment 75
 Chapter 6: Human Emotions 77
  Listen to Your Emotions 81
  Polarity 84
  Let it Flow 87
  HEART: Human Experience 90
PART 4: RESILIENCE 91
 Chapter 7: The "D" Word 93
  "F" Words 97
  What's in Your Backpack? 98
  Forgiveness 100
  LOVE 104
  HEART: Unpack Your Backpack 105
 Chapter 8: Another "F" Word 107
  If You're Not Growing, You're Shrinking 109
  From the Mouths of Babes… 110
  F*CK IT… 112
  HEART: Cuts Like a Knife 115
  HEART: Word to the Words 117
PART 5: TRUST 119
 Chapter 9: The 3Ms 121
  Mindfulness 123
  Movement 126

  Marijuana 128
   HEART: Mind & Body 133
   HEART: Never Have I Ever 134
 Chapter 10: Helping Hands 137
  Who Are You? 140
  What Do You Need? 145
  Help Yourself 146
   HEART: Self Care 148
PART 6: H.E.A.R.T. 149
 Chapter 11: The 4th "M" is Magic 151
  Messages & Gifts 152
  Animals 154
  Spirituality 156
  Full Circle 158
  The Voice Within 161
   Daily Practices 162
   HEART: Ho'oponopono 164
   HEART: Authentic Self 166
 Chapter 12: Heart First 167
  "You Cannot Truly Love Others, Until You Love Yourself" 169
   Connect 170
  Tune In 172
  Trust your Gut, Destiny, Life, Karma, Whatever ... 175
   HUMAN 176
   EMPOWERMENT 177
   ALIGNMENT 177
   RESILIENCE 177
   TRUST 178
   HEART: Love Yourself 180

- Conclusion 181
  - Bonus Chapter: Twin Flame 185
    - Manifest Destiny 188
    - Lighting the Fire 191
    - Magic, Miracles, & Love 193
    - Second Attempt 196
    - Law of Attraction 200
      - HEART: Twin Flames 202
- Nancy Seibel 203
  - The Nancy Perspective 203
    - Qualifications 205
    - Get in Touch 205
- Resources 207

Introduction

I have one mission with this book: To wake you up to the magic that comes with self love and help you find your way back to your HEART.

Underneath all the pain you have endured, the sadness you have held and the numbing you didn't even know you were doing, is a person worth believing in again.

Trust me. I know this deep down in my soul because I have been you.

I lost myself in sickness. I lost myself because I tried to take on the world and conquer it like the warrior I was, and I failed miserably. To date, this has become my greatest blessing.

For I, like many of us, was on a path of destruction towards money, power, and "keeping up with the Joneses" to the point that I almost did not have a life to keep up with anymore.

I was SUPERHUMAN in all aspects of my life...I was at the top of my game in work, life, and play, and it appeared like I had it all together. And yet, underneath it all, I was withering away little by little.

My blessing came 8 years ago when my mom dragged me to a very reputable hospital in the U.S., thinking I was dying, to find out it was ONLY chronic fatigue syndrome (CFS) and fibromyalgia (FIBRO). I had pushed my body to its limits and had no choice but to find a way to do it all differently.

I was on 10 pills a day when I arrived at the hospital. Since then, I have eliminated all of them except my thyroid pills. For 3 years, I was on 100 mg a day of an antidepressant, and now the only thing I require is a few puffs of weed at night to help me sleep.

My wake-up call is my greatest blessing—not because it has not been easy healing from the inside out, but because it was what I needed to wake me up to what I had been missing out on—ME.

Would you be surprised to know that finding my way back to self love (HEART), from the inside out, was my greatest healing ever out of FIBRO and CFS?

Not only did it heal me, but its power also healed the 2 most important people in my world—my daughters. When we choose to heal ourselves from the inside out, we become a mirror that guides others to do the same, especially those who are close to our hearts. The more I healed and embraced the happiness and self love within, the more I saw it happening within my girls too and that has brought me to a place I never imagined.

What if, through seeking self love, one small step at a time (vs. the all or nothing mentality we have all tried to embrace), we can unravel all the anger, sadness, ho hum, etc. we hold within and start to shift it all.

It starts with choosing you.

Take a small step every single day (regardless of how small the step is) and celebrate each one, MOMENT BY MOMENT, STEP BY STEP.

You know how much you love your kids? Your dog? You know what you would do for them to keep them happy? What if today, all you did was take some of that love you so easily give to others and shift it back to you. A little at a time. A small step at a time.

What if, while you do this, you also choose to start seeing things differently? You choose to slowly start to shift your perspective out of your head and into your heart, out of overthinking and towards the love and compassion you so easily share with others. Not to reduce the love we give to others, but to increase our capacity for love.

Perspective is our greatest choice forward. Perspective has the power to change everything. Regardless of what happens, how you see it can either force you deeper into the hole or empower you to rise above, and it all comes down to a simple shift in thinking. PERSPECTIVE and SMALL STEPS FORWARD.

True, you will not be perfect at this, and you will fail daily—however, the lessons you learn as you fail may just empower you to keep pushing. I am 8 years into shifting my perspective moment by moment and making small steps daily towards self love, and the magic surrounding me is incredible!

As I have healed, I continue to grow and learn and do it all with love and compassion wrapped around my soul. I am far from perfect and f*ck up often, however, when I do, I remind myself to wrap all the love I so easily give away around me, knowing I have the choice to try again in the next moment.

I have lost everything on my journey back to self love (HEART)—my career path, my marriage, my old self. I've gained happiness and peace from the inside out, and what I see in my kids—kindness, compassion, and love—tells me that regardless of the pain I have felt, I am on the right path forward.

Choosing me. Choosing happiness. Choosing my HEART. Why do I capitalize HEART, you ask? It's become a way of life for me, and my hope is that it becomes the same for you…as you unravel, empower, and believe in YOU again.

Your time is NOW. Trust me. What you believe in yourself to be true, is true, and today is the DAY to make the choice to start living your self again, moment by moment, choice by choice, and perspective by perspective.

You are so worthy of this shift and now, more than ever, the world is asking you to do so. WE must choose our HEART because love that is cultivated from the inside out has the power to create all that you have ever desired.

You are one small step away. Stop telling yourself otherwise. You are so worthy of healing, change, and love.

Nancy

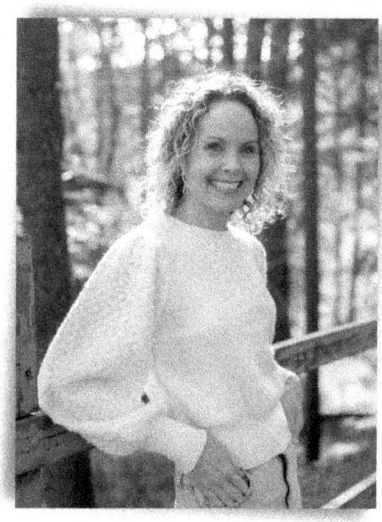

Photo Credit: Jenny Scott

PLEASE NOTE: All of my words come from 2 places—love and faith. I am no scientist and the knowledge I've acquired is self taught through certifications and my own experience. These words are my OPINIONs backed by experience and knowledge with a hope to empower you. Believe and trust that you are way more powerful than the world has led you to believe. I believe we are being asked to tune in and open our minds to our most powerful opportunity to move forward.

Part 1: Human

Chapter 1: The Universe Keeps Knocking

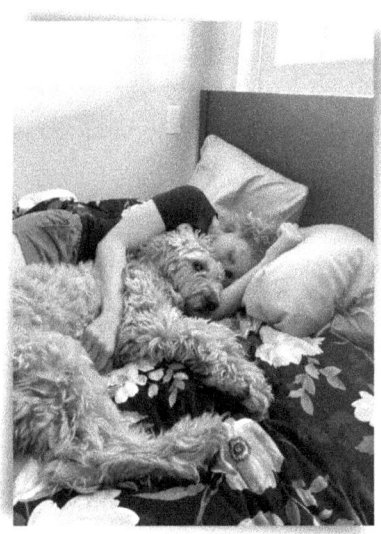

In 2015, I ended up at a very reputable hospital in the U.S. I now know, looking back, that this was the moment in time that shifted my entire soul forward.

Up until 2015, I was living my life like society asks us to. I wanted to fit in. I wanted to show the world I could do it too. So, when I met an incredible man in 2005, I jumped in. By 2006, we moved in together and in 2008, we were married. Our children followed in 2009/2011. In 2012, I started back to work and my goal was "to get to the top." I was ready to show the world the superhuman that was Nancy F*CKing Seibel.

I laugh as I write this…despite the fact that I was trying so hard to fit in and do everything, the universe had different plans for me…

I was a "fake it 'til I make it" type of girl. I was taught early in life that if you show up confidently and keep learning, you can do and be anything. The greatest wake-up call came when I realized I could not do it anymore because of my health.

I am amazed, looking back, at how invincible we as HUMANS really are and yet…

We Can Only Go So Far

By the time 2015 hit, I had conquered and built an amazing life that looked incredible on social media. On the inside, I had nothing left. I was numb. And, more importantly, I wasn't listening. My body was stockpiling sickness. Underneath the authentic positivity of Nancy, I was losing my power within.

I was on edge all the time…I felt almost as though I was running a marathon daily since my body never stopped feeling anxious. There were days that all I could do was get my kids to school and then come home to do nothing. There were days that the pain was so unbearable, I found myself lying in bed, unable to do much more than wonder what the f*ck was going on. There were days that no matter how much I pushed to get myself moving, my body clearly said "F*CK no!" The energy I used to have wasn't showing up anymore, and I kept pushing…but I wasn't capable of pushing beyond it.

My body had symptom after symptom…stomach issues, acid reflux, chronic pain, heart palpitations, my right side even stopped working at one point…it was numb.

In the first 6 months after my first daughter was born, I was up every night all night long. I couldn't sleep at all, regardless of the medication I was given. My body was supposed to be in "fully functioning" mode and yet, I knew I wasn't.

I could sense I was losing myself slowly…I started to no longer care about the things I used to…how clean my house was…showing up perfect…the cracks just started happening and I didn't know what to do to slow them down.

My children started to yell and cry daily, and my body started to wither away and yell louder and louder. By the time I ended up at the hospital, I was sick and yet still fully functioning. My thyroid had been so high and my body so off that I should have been hospitalized, yet I was still SHOWING up: At work, at CrossFit, and at HOME.

I became a hypochondriac, but I knew deep down I wasn't well. I am blessed by my Mom. She saw what I was attempting to carry and knew that if she didn't get me help, I wouldn't make it in this world.

After 5 years of weekly doctor's appointments, multiple tests which showed nothing, and pill after pill for symptoms that manifested even more symptoms, my mom and I had had enough of the medical system and went to the US for help. That week at the hospital is why I am still here and begging you to listen.

That week I wasn't given a diagnosis of death. I was given a diagnosis of opportunity— FIBRO-F*CKING-MYALGIA and CHRONIC FATIGUE SYNDROME…and a huge opportunity to shift it all. I was given a choice that day and words that resonated in my soul that I've carried with me since.

THERE IS NO YOU, WITHOUT YOU

The words from the doctor that day started, "There is no you, without you." It went on. "You are welcome to go HOME and continue on this path you are on. If you do though, I am NOT sure you will come back here next year. OR you can go home, PAUSE it all, UNRAVEL it all, and REWIRE it all.

You have kids at home who need you to be here. You have a job you've chosen to prioritize. You are attempting to "keep up with the Joneses." And it's killing you…

You must STOP. And the only person who's going to make you do that...is you. This choice all comes back to YOU."

I wasn't prescribed more meds that day, however, what I was prescribed, shifted it all—REST, MINDFULNESS, and a FULL STOP.

I remember being told to go home, put on my housecoat, and watch a full series of a show on the couch. This was something I had NO Idea how to do...

I was a triple type A personality with a drive and determination that allowed me to push through anything and now I was being asked to stop...FULL F*CKING STOP.

WTF. I am invincible! I can fight and push through anything...

- I don't have PTSD.
- I don't have ANXIETY.
- I don't have work to do on MYSELF.
- This is everyone else's fault.
- I am amazing the way I am.
- I am a fighter and can conquer anything.

- I am FINE.

WTF!

BAHAHAHAHAHAHAHHAHAHA...

...Until You Listen

That day, I chose to go home and make a decision that shifted my whole life. I quit my job, walked away from all the plans I'd had, and made it a mission to learn how to do life differently...I chose to put every ounce of effort I had easily given to others back on myself. To learn how to embrace the things I was so afraid of and learn how to use the powerful tools of mindfulness and rewiring that I'd been taught...the most important lesson I learned that day was to stop fighting myself and start loving myself.

F**********CK!

HEART: 180 Degrees

Where does your story begin? Have you received a diagnosis of some sort? Have you received a wake-up call? If you were to complete the following statement, what would it say: Everything was going according to plan until…

_____
_____
_____
_____
_____
_____
_____
_____
_____
_____

Chapter 2: What is Your Body Trying to Tell You?

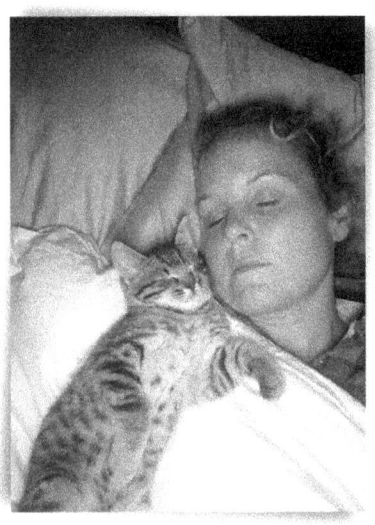

I spent most of my career in pharma, believing in the power of medicine and pills. I was a science girl. I was a girl who didn't believe in "woo woo" things...and yet, by the time I was 35, I was on a different pill for every different symptom I had. The pills were part of the reason I ended up being as sick as I was. Since my visit to the hospital and since learning differently, my entire way of feeling and healing has changed.

What if you knew that pain wasn't just your body's way of yelling at you or trying desperately to get your attention, but a huge opportunity to unravel what you are attempting to numb?

What if you knew that pain was there to guide you, back within your body. What if you realized that your body was trying to help you "feel" again and that by ignoring it, the pain only gets louder, stronger, and more painful?

What is incredible to me is that "feelings" aren't really being felt by people. It's why pain and chronic illness are on the rise, now more than ever. We are so NUMB to all that has happened that we've chosen to ignore the more important aspect of being HUMAN—emotions. In the next few years, I predict a huge amount of physical illness related to emotional pain.

I know how pain feels. I am "blessed" to wake up daily not yet knowing the pain I will feel that day.

Some days my entire right side does not function properly. Some days I can complete a CrossFit workout almost Rx (at the athlete level), and some days I can only do body weight. As a result of ignoring my pain for so long, I am now "blessed" to have messages of pain daily to remind me that I still have work to do. The pain used to control me, it used to make me hide from the world and feel scared of everything. If you knew me 10 years ago, you'd know me as the extrovert who thrived on having humans around to function (my numbing technique), but now, I am more of a hermit because I choose to take the time I need to listen to what my beautiful body is trying to tell me and do things differently.

From Numb, to Pain, and Beyond

What if...

- pain is our way to tune in?

- pain is really an emotion we are choosing to block?
- illness is our opportunity to really pay attention to what our body has been trying to tell us for so long that now it's yelling?
- you knew that according to science, 98% of illnesses are energetically related (epigenetics)?[1]
- you knew that if you tuned into the pain you are being asked to feel, and understood the emotions related to that pain, you could slowly start to unravel the pain and actually heal?

I've done this. Over and over, and as a result, not only does the pain NOT define me anymore, but there are also many days that I have NO pain. As I've learned to unravel the pain, I've studied this incredible opportunity we have as HUMANS right now.

Louise Hay has been one of my guides. She is the author of so many incredible books related to

---

[1] Lipton, B. (2021). The Power of Consciousness. Interview by Iain McNay. Retrieved from https://conscious.tv/text/53.htm

matching pain with emotions and guiding us with affirmations to unravel them.

I know this sounds crazy and yet the field of epigenetics (new science in the last 50 years) supports this information and is proving that HUMANs are way more f*cking powerful then we ever knew we were.[2]

Back to the 98 percent...here is what we are learning from a scientific perspective. We used to think that the body only existed as a physical entity, which meant we needed to rely on physical medicine to heal. We get sick, we go to the doctor for medicine, and we heal. That's why I was on 10 pills a day—to heal. What I am seeing now, because scientists have chosen to reconnect with the energetic perspective of the body (first through quantum physics and now epigenetics), is that we are more energetically aligned than physically aligned which means there is HUGE potential in what we can discover around self healing.

---

[2] Spinney, L. (2021, Oct. 10). Epigenetics, the misunderstood science that could shed new light on ageing. *The Guardian*. Retrieved from https://www.theguardian.com/science/2021/oct/10/epigenetics-the-misunderstood-science-that-could-shed-new-light-on-ageing

Misalignment

Everything in this world is energy. Powerful swirls of mini tornados that come together and form physical spaces. In our incredible bodies, energy is controlled by our hearts and our hearts read energy by way of emotions. Our hearts start beating long before anything else in our vessel, and they really are the key to unlocking it all. Our hearts are guided by emotions, and the emotions we feel control the environments of our bodies. Every emotion creates hormones and reactions that flow through our body. What is released based on the emotion we feel is how our bodies choose to react. If you are in a constant overthinking victim mentality, you are constantly creating an environment that is full of the same, and the hormones that get released are a result of the emotions you feel (stress hormones, etc.). If you are holding space for love, feeling joy, and cultivating positivity daily, the environment that flows through your body matches your vibes and optimal health usually follows. Here is the caveat—you cannot fool your body. The body knows when the words and energy are misaligned, and it will keep yelling until you choose to align them. It's why words and thoughts are way more powerful than HUMANS choose to believe, and it's why I now "yell" self love to myself and others daily.

For a long time, I used positivity on the outside and felt negative thoughts within. This is why I ended up with fibromyalgia. According to Louise Hay, fibromyalgia is a dissonance of your soul—a disconnect between your inner and outer thoughts.[3] The flow and the hormones in my body matched the inner words and feelings I felt and therefore, over time, the pain built up. Now, as I've really understood and implemented the incredible wisdom of Louise Hay as my guide (and the supporting science), I've unravelled the pain, shifted my inner thoughts, rewired my brain through mindfulness, and connected back to the positive force that I am—INSIDE and OUT. Over time, this shift has also shifted my body...out of survival mode and into something I never imagined possible again. THRIVING.

This transformation hasn't been easy and it's often a moment-by-moment assessment to keep myself aligned, but what it's done is magical. It's why I yell

---

[3] Hay, L. (1984, Jan. 1). *Heal Your Body: The Mental Causes for Physical Illness and the Metaphysical Way to Overcome Them.* Hay House, Inc.

SELF LOVE so freaking loud. The more I've learned to truly and authentically love myself—through words, affirmations, and trust—the more I've healed within. The way I've done all my healing is not through doctors and medicine but by unravelling all the things I chose to ignore. I faced all the things I didn't love about myself and chose to fall in love all over again.

I am no longer on 10 pills a day...I am now on one pill a day and that pill is for my thyroid. Some people call me superhuman because I've even cut my dose of thyroid medicine in half this past year as a result of the energetic healing work I've done. When I am "blessed" with a FIBRO flare up, I use it as an opportunity to tune into what my body is trying to tell me and give it the time it needs to rest and heal. These are the times I now go inward, hermit and use my love as my superpower to heal. You have this same POWER.

If you had known me before and seen me after, you'd see the amazing work I've done and know that there is truth in the things I am saying.

So here is my ask...tune in!

Empower Yourself

Stop believing everything you've been told and open your mind:

1. Go to the doctor and understand what the pain is trying to tell you through bloodwork, etc. You must know what you are facing in order to empower and heal.
2. Get the diagnosis, take the pills...hear what they are saying, however, DO NOT accept this as the only way forward.
3. Find an energetic healer and open your mind to the awareness of what is possible beyond what you've been taught to think.
4. Look up LOUISE HAY and her wisdoms: and START saying them out loud...and find a way of FEELING it... https://www.louisehay.com
5. Look up EPIGENETICS and start taking the steps you need towards a different path. Bruce Lipton is a good starting place: https://www.brucelipton.com

And more importantly than ever, believe that you are more f*cking powerful than we've ever been taught to believe.

What's crazy to me is that those of us who already know what I am preaching are the ones who have had to experience a powerful wake-up call. Now I'm begging all of you to pause and tune into the powerful force that we are as HUMANS with ENERGY.

We are all superhuman. We are all capable of so much more than you ever imagined...all you gotta do is choose to do it differently and start right now.

Open your mind...the time is now my friend...what are you waiting for???

HEART: Listen to Your Body

What physical nudges have you experienced repeatedly/ongoing or are you experiencing now that might be trying to tell you something? What other message could you be missing? If your back hurts, perhaps you're feeling the betrayal of a friend. If you're having issues with your lungs, perhaps you're feeling the weight of your commitments. If you've lost your voice or your throat hurts, maybe you feel as though your voice isn't being heard. List them out so you can refer back to them as you read the rest of the book!

_____
_____
_____
_____
_____
_____
_____
_____
_____
_____
_____

Part 2: Empowerment

Chapter 3: My Unravelling

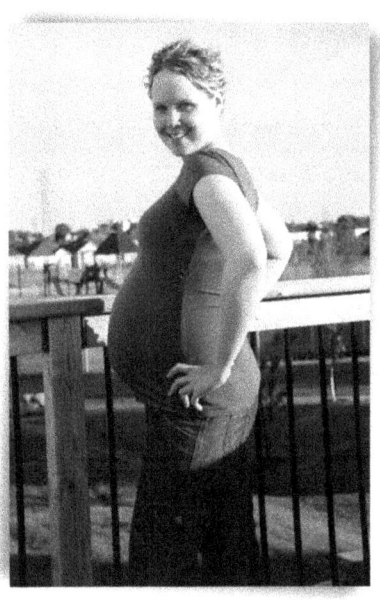

I was a girl with a vision, a plan, a girl who knew where she was going, who had her sh*t together and that people looked up to…I had it all. I went out and chose well and felt like I was on top of the world…until it all came crashing down—little by little—just after I had children.

> If you're anything like me, you may have had a "June Cleaver" mom. It was wonderful. The unconditional love, patience, and warmth flowing from this pure spirit was amazing.
>
> But...it set an impossible motherhood standard. Impossible standards are everywhere around us. The words "hustle," fight, push...these words are not what we are meant to embody. The energy of who you are within is who you should become outwardly.
>
> If you push through and embody the "hustle" outwardly, it creeps in and challenges the energy of who you are actually meant to be.
>
>

Superwoman

I went out and did everything society told me to do and thought I was doing it right. I bought into the "dream" and subscribed to the formula...

- Go to university

- Get a good job
- Find a man
- Get married
- Find a home
- Have children

It's all a race to have children. Society tells you that if you aren't married or have a house or career, you don't have kids. So, the race is on to find that person and do all the things to get to having children if you want them.

The problem is that you might be picking the wrong person, the wrong career, the wrong house but not even realize it until your biggest challenge comes along…kids. Then you have to unravel the pieces because it's the wrong combination, and the tearing down and rebuilding is so much harder.

All these things did was push me further away from who I was meant to be, and my many wake-up calls were the moments in time when I needed to pay attention versus keep pushing forward.

The baby boomer generation was also the beginning of moms working. They went back to work or they worked all along. But they kept up with the domestic duties too. We were socialized by superwomen to DO IT ALL.

In trying to be like our moms, we hustle, we don't give up, we don't even stop because if we stop then we're not living up to the standard. Is it ridiculous to try? Absolutely. Do we do it anyways? Absolutely. We wanted to be them. And we wanted to be them so badly that we don't know who we are.

We tried so hard to meet and surpass their "success" because we wanted to make them proud. It's so wonderful to have such a stellar role model, but it sets the bar high. And they were conditioned by society to set their bar…and the cycle goes on and on.

Here's the bottom line—there's a disconnect between what our parents did and what we need to do…so to force yourself to keep on fighting the fight and doing it the way they did will get you nowhere. You are your own person and you need to listen to your HEART and the hearts of your children.

Great "Mom" Expectations

Nobody tells you how hard it is to have kids. But if someone were to try to tell you...would you believe them? No. It's a reality that you have to experience to know. You are supposed to love your children immediately after you have them. You are supposed to have a maternal instinct to care for your child. Mothering is supposed to come naturally. It's supposed to be the most wonderful time in your life. It's a f*cking sh*t show.

In 2009 upon the delivery of my first beautiful girl, I was blessed with a "f*ck up" in the delivery room that shifted it all. I arrived that day at the hospital very excited about my daughter being brought into this world. I had my nails done, hair done, and remembered joking about how beautiful I looked. My expectation was smooth sailing - that it would all happen with ease and I'd go home into the fairytale world I still believed in.

After check in, the normal routine followed suit and just before delivery, it all went to sh*t. They made a mistake in my bloodwork, which caused all of us (doctor and nurses included) to believe there was a chance I wasn't going to make it out of the delivery room. They were worried about me hemorrhaging, and when my daughter's heart rate dropped, they coded me.

The sh*tty thing about being coded that day was that I knew too much and, when I heard it, I knew it wasn't good. I watched as the doctor's face went GRAY and my mom, who had been sitting in the corner, was now standing up SCARED as HELL. We both thought I was going to die. I still cry when I think about that moment. All I remember thinking is "don't take me...please don't take me." The only thing I ever wanted was to be a MOM and, in that moment, there was a chance it was going to be taken away. But then came the moment that really shifted it all.

Just after Lucy was born and the bloodwork was repeated, we learned it was all a mistake...a f*cking mistake...and yet that moment was now imprinted in my soul so deeply that I wasn't sure I'd ever feel the same again. As a result, my beautiful daughter was born into this world and I felt NOTHING. PTSD hit hard after that and instead of pausing to tune in, I kept moving forward. A diagnosis of Hashimoto's (thyroid) soon followed and yet I chose to keep showing up because I had to be a MOM.

I remember coming home from the hospital after having my first daughter and being completely lost. I remember the first 24 hours almost as a blur because I didn't know how to breastfeed. I was scared sh*tless. I remember sitting on the couch for the first 3 months staring at my dining room table thinking... *is this it?*

I had plans on how to be a mom and that all changed in the delivery room that day. I went home numb, and after that I went mechanical and just tried to still be a good mom without feeling. My daughter could tell. I had trouble breastfeeding—I hired an expert breastfeeding nurse for 3 hours and she told me to quit because it was causing too much stress. I started learning a very powerful lesson that day about the mirror reflection—everything I felt, my daughter felt, and if I was stressed while I was feeding her, she too was stressed trying to eat. I didn't know that everything I felt, my kids felt...

We had our first child in Oshawa, Ontario and moved to Halifax, Nova Scotia within the first year of her life. It took me about 2 years to get pregnant the first time and I had to go on medication in order for it to happen but the second time, it was immediate. Funny how overthinking it the first time around was actually a hindrance.

It is wild that there is no education on how to be a parent. I had this plan of how it was going to go...and yet it all went to sh*t. There is no one that tells you that becoming a mom takes your entire old life away and demands that you surrender control...the more control I tried to have, the more lost I felt and the more afraid I was of losing control. There is no one that tells us how to go back to work after becoming a mom, or how to keep up the same driven mentality while raising children. I would go to work everyday, kick a**, and come home to tired kids who just wanted their mom and I was so tired...

Every time I see a young mom now, I am drawn to them. I now go up to them to tell them how amazing they are, even if I don't know them. I always take the time to remind them of their awesomeness. I always say, "I drank a lot, I cried a lot, and I sat in the corner a lot and said WTF."

A Dose of Reality

In the first 5 years of both my daughters' lives, after sending them to daycare they were sick at least 2 of the 5 days. I would have to leave work, take time off, or work from home. At that time, it was still looked down upon if I stayed home but I had no choice.

My kids also cried every single time they got in the car…the entire car ride…I used to cry with them. Our "natural" bond was hindered because of my PTSD—and my daughter felt it–she would cry every time she got tired as she didn't know how to self soothe. Often, she would rage and I would have to sit in her room for hours with her until she calmed. I had to learn to become calm even in my chaos.

At my worst I used to listen to 680 news all day long, then sit in the car and do a meditation to try and prepare myself for parenting. But I would come in the house and it would be a mess from the morning and I would lose it. It was too much. In response, my kids would throw stuff at me all night long. You keep doing what society says you should do as a parent, but it doesn't work. You're still striving for the June Cleaver standard which is impossible.

There is a book on trauma by Gabor Mate, *The Myth of Normal,*[4] which talks about why kids have trauma and I checked all the boxes for both my girls right from the start. You are pretty much failing everyday as a mom. If I failed, I walked away, started again, and moved forward—but you can't do this while being a mom...trust me, I tried. I even got to the point when I consciously chose work first because I felt I had failed so badly. I was watching my family fall apart and it was easier to step out of it rather than face it...

The hardest part of being a parent is watching everything you dislike about yourself come out in your children...every emotion you've tried to hide comes out ready to be faced...they truly show you both the best and the worst of yourself. There is no one to tell you that these beautiful children are your mirror reflections. There is no one that tells you how to work together in having kids.

My unravelling involved analyzing many aspects of my life. It started externally with things and people I brought into my life, with evaluating what society tells

---

[4] Mate, G. (2022, Sept. 12). *The Myth of Normal: Trauma, Illness and Healing in a Toxic Culture.* Knopf Canada.

us, and trying to find my own version of happiness within society's structure. Eventually though, my unravelling led me to analyze myself, who I had become and who I really wanted and needed to be. Unravelling isn't a process of falling apart, it's a process of pulling apart with intention to discover the truth. It's letting go of control and feeling uncomfortable. And it's ongoing. There is always more to learn, you are never finished. The answers come from inside of you, not outside.

HEART: Superpower Playlist

MUSIC was one of my superpowers throughout all this, I used to make my children watch music videos and just sing a lot...to keep myself sane. "Good Life" by OneRepublic was the song I would put on every time people were crying in my house and then everyone would stop crying. Like within 2 minutes...to this day it still has the same effect. In my house, we often have dance parties. It immediately shifts the energy in the room, even in the hardest of times.

You can do it too...what songs immediately put a smile on your face and make you want to sing and dance. List them below and create a superpower playlist!

_____

_____

_____

_____

_____

_____

_____

_____

_____

HEART: Great Expectations

What expectations did you have before you started your career, marriage, parenting, or other life journey? How have those expectations changed? What advice would you give someone about to embark on that same/similar journey? How can you repurpose that advice for yourself?

_____

_____

_____

_____

_____

_____

_____

_____

_____

_____

_____

Chapter 4: Do it For You AND Your Family

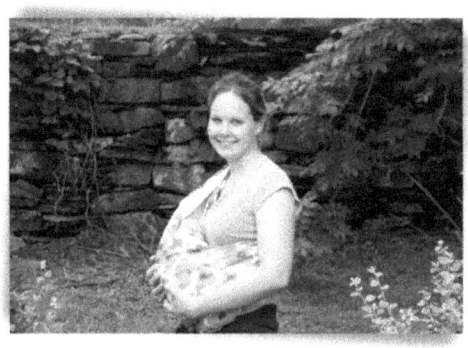

What if your kids aren't thriving because deep down you aren't either? What if your kids are the key to unlocking the emotions you hold within, and all you've got to do right now is lean in and observe? What if you are about to stop reading because you "feel" you aren't NUMB, and yet your kids are yelling in a way you've never seen before? What if you don't have to feel guilty but can instead become empowered as a parent and take the next step, right now?

I am sitting back, reading all about the unbelievable chaos that our children are experiencing and it's igniting a frustration in me that I need to share.

My parenting wake-up call came when my girls were 2 and 4. I was attempting to take on the world and be a superhero in all aspects of my life, and I was failing miserably. I was rocking it in my career and failing in the place that mattered most—at home. I was faking it all and hoping that like everything else...if I faked it, I'd eventually make it. I was NUMBING it all and hoping "it" would pass.

My kids were yelling every day and despite the fact I was using calming tools to shift my energy, they saw through it all and showed up in a way that I had NO IDEA HOW TO DEAL WITH. So, we visited a counsellor for help. We sat in an office for about $5,000 worth of counselling, and no kids were ever included. It was becoming clear to me that I needed the courage to ask a very powerful question that I had been avoiding and yet, I knew I needed to hear the answer.

> Why aren't my kids here? We are hoping to get guidance and help with our kids, however, they aren't here for you to observe and assess??? Why not?
>
> The answer that came that day shifted my entire life…
>
>

The Mirror

I admit that in that moment, I cowered with guilt, shame, sadness, and fear as she spoke the words: YOUR KIDS ARE A MIRROR REFLECTION OF YOU.

Kids are superpower feelers and their abilities to show you your own emotions are incredible. All you've got to do as a parent is TUNE in, observe how they are showing up, and use this as your guide to move forward.

WHAT? I am not angry! I am not crying endlessly! I am not screaming and looking at myself with such frustration and anger! WTF???????

The next thing she said blew my mind.

"What if you are? What if, underneath the way you 'think' you are showing up, is actually the truth and you've NUMBED it all because it's the only coping strategy you've been taught? What if, the best way forward isn't to attempt to fix your children, but instead DIVE deep into yourself and face the emotions you've been NUMBING your entire life?"

You have no idea the spiral downward that came after this moment. I didn't believe her, so I went home and did research of my own only to find out that SHE WAS SPOT ON.

Epigenetics

The science that backs this claim is incredible:

> "All of us got programmed the first seven years of our life. We play the program 95 percent of the day," Lipton said. "The conscious mind, which is the creator mind, is separate from the subconscious mind, which is the programmed mind. The significance is that subconscious is on autopilot, and if 95

percent of your life is coming from the subconscious, then you are playing programs and you're not playing creator. The issue is the programs we got in the first seven years, up to 60 percent of those programs are beliefs, they're things that are disempowering, they're self-sabotaging, or limiting behaviors, and therefore, we're losing power in the program that says, 'Who do you think you are? You don't deserve that. You're not that smart.' These are things we acquired when we were young."[5]

There is so much to learn in those first 7 years of life that nature actually intuitively aligns us with those around us to become our greatest mirrors. Who are those people? Our parents, our friends, the environments in which we function. The ways they are taught to cope, the ways they love, and the ways they treat others are all a reflection of the things we've taught them, unconsciously as their parents. It is only after the age of 8 that their brains shift into another state and this state opens the door to perspective. As we all know, perspective only develops over time with life lessons and awareness, and this process takes a lifetime.

---

[5] Gutshtein, N. (2022, May 29). Dr. Bruce Lipton Reacts to New Map of Human Genome. *Gaia: Transformation, Alternative Health, Secrets To Health*. Retrieved from https://www.gaia.com/article/dr-bruce-lipton-reacts-to-new-map-of-human-genome

UGH...

The reflection I saw of the 2 young girls SCREAMING at me daily was SO HARD TO see and accept, but I know all of this to be true...because almost 6 years later, the reflection I now see as a result of this profound awareness is why I need you to hear what I'm yelling.

YOU have CHOICE only in the NOW.

Go Inward

We cannot look back and stay too long in the guilt we are choosing to hold as a result of this awareness. We must see the opportunity in what is being asked and move forward knowing we are the key to unlocking it all. So, if your kids are:

- Giving you dirty looks...
- NOT talking about their emotions...
- Talking unkindly of others...
- Judging others...
- Focusing too much on their looks...
- Having perfection issues...
- Anger issues...
- Anxiety issues...

- Too much technology…
- Distraction issues…

Here is your parenting WAKE-UP CALL. STOP BLAMING YOUR KIDS. STOP TRYING TO FIX YOUR KIDS. START becoming aware of your greatest opportunity right now for you and your family, YOUR OWN GROWTH.

If you are choosing to raise your children as your parents did and not adapting to the ever-changing world around us, your children will continue on the same path and barely survive in this world.

It's time we did it differently. What is the greatest gift that happens as a result? We start to feel in little moments. You have to let yourself feel, which is an act of self love. The logic in your brain keeps trying to rationalize, but you have to let the feelings come out as uncomfortable as they might be. The emotions are uncomfortable because you don't have control, but the point is to let go and keep letting go. And as I went inward and felt through the NUMBNESS I created, what came was a newfound love of flow, of trust, and of intuitive guidance, and more importantly a newfound love of myself.

When we love ourselves and strive for happiness within, we show our kids they are worthy of the same. You have this same choice…trust me…the time is NOW.

Mirror mirror on the wall,
You have the choice to shift it all.
Follow the path back towards you,
and watch magic happen in all that you do.
Our kids are the reason we must choose to thrive,
Now, more than ever, they need us to guide.
We only have "choice," right now, in the now…
So, choose to grow, shift, and change, and be open to "wow"!

HEART: Look in the Mirror

What are the things that you see in your children which you would like to change? Where in your life do you see that behaviour, from yourself or other key members of your children's family or support network? What behaviour would you like them to demonstrate instead and how can you use that to adjust your approach as a parent?

_____
_____
_____
_____
_____
_____
_____
_____
_____
_____
_____

HEART: Tune In

Find a comfortable, quiet spot to sit down. Close your eyes. Start by noticing what you can hear. What background noises do you notice? Then notice what you can smell. What do you feel? Your clothes on your skin, the chair underneath you? Now what do you feel inside your body? How do your muscles feel? Are you relaxed? Now what emotions do you feel? Where are these emotions coming from? Ask the question, but if the answer doesn't come, don't worry…it will.

_____

_____

_____

_____

_____

_____

_____

_____

_____

_____

_____

Part 3: Alignment

Chapter 5: The BIG Job

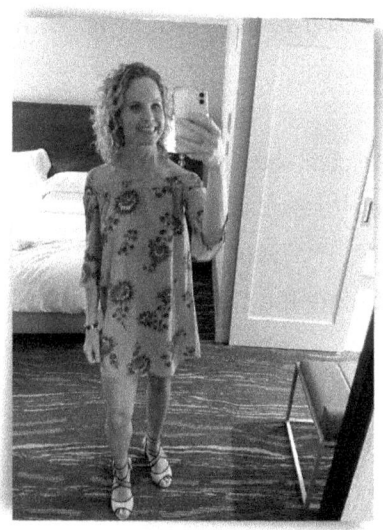

What pisses me off about the world is that we're taught to fight our own nature. Why? Because you need to be a functioning, contributing member of society? Because there's no profit to be made by having a world full of healthy, happy people? Because we live in a patriarchal society, and the image of a man has been hyper masculine, money making, successful, and powerful?

> That's why we keep emotion out of business. Or we did, until women entered the workforce. Women were raised differently from men. But men have an unravelling of their own to do as a result of their conditioning.
>
> The victim mentality is conveniently provided by society to explain why you aren't happy with the life they've told you to create. It tells you that other people are the cause of your discontent or making you live a certain way. But here's the thing...you always have a CHOICE in YOU. No one is making you do anything...
>
>

The Dream

We try to listen to the lessons of our parents and apply them to our lives. What is the secret to their perceived success? If you go out and get THE BIG JOB, you can have it all. But if someone tried to tell you that making it to the top was overrated, you wouldn't believe them.

The trifecta: job, marriage, children. You can't rock them all at the same time. One has to fall.

Maybe for our parents it didn't happen right away, maybe it didn't happen at all in the public eye. But their marriages fail, they hate their jobs, they struggle with parenthood. It's behind the scenes because they don't "air out their dirty laundry."

We can't keep racing towards a finish line that isn't our own. I'm not talking about the difference between a job in one industry versus another. I'm not talking about having 2 kids or 3. We have the power to design our own lives and it doesn't have to follow the formula…

Set Up to Fail

I always wanted to be a really good mom. I wanted the perfect family, the perfect husband for children, and the perfect career path. I wanted it all and thought that I could achieve it, like Cinderella did, in a way that would be exactly what I planned. My mom did everything for us to make sure that our lives were different than hers. My mom was my role model in everything I did and, like so many of us, we push forward on the path our parents want for us versus the path we want to take. That's where challenges often start to present themselves.

I have already mentioned that epigenetics states by the age of 7, 90% of our programming is ingrained in our brain.[6] This means most of us are programmed by our parents because we are mere reflections of them until the age of 8. After the age of 8 up to 25 (mostly for men) we learn perspective, and through perspective we start to navigate our lives in the way that we as human beings want. Learning this powerful information made me wake up to so many moments in my life where my path went wrong. When I look back now, I realize that the first 8 years of my life were not easy. I experienced my parents' divorce at the age of 2. I watched my mom be sad and have to rebuild her life in a way that makes me super proud, however, as a child I also felt everything she did on top of carrying my own. I also carried her pain and sadness as I tried to navigate the world. Kids are

---

[6] Gustafson, C., Lipton, B. (2017, Dec.). The Jump From Cell Culture to Consciousness. *Integr Med (Encinitas)*, 16(6). Pp. 44-50. PMID: 30936816; PMCID: PMC6438088. Retrieved from https://www.ncbi.nlm.nih.gov/pmc/articles/PMC6438088/; Gutshtein, N. (2022, May 29). Dr. Bruce Lipton Reacts to New Map of Human Genome. *Gaia: Transformation, Alternative Health, Secrets To Health.* Retrieved from https://www.gaia.com/article/dr-bruce-lipton-reacts-to-new-map-of-human-genome

feelers in this world and my greatest wake-up call in my whole life was recognizing how much of my family dynamic I have been carrying as an adult and that has affected my entire life.

What I was taught as a child was not wrong or right, however, my mom always taught us to be independent, strong, financially-stable women. As a result, my path forward was all about money. I can see that clearly now, but at the time I only knew that I was driven and ready to conquer the world, doing what society told me to do. I remember coming out of University and getting my first job in the publishing industry. I was 22 years old and I was making $41,000 a year. At the same time, my sister started in a pharmaceutical job and she was making $80,000 a year. During those first 2 years as a publishing rep, I rocked my career, became Rookie of the Year, and unravelled many impossible standards to become what I wanted to be...which was the best in everything I did. Once I proved to myself that I could do and be what I wanted to be, I left the publishing industry (even though it was a passion of mine) and chose to go into pharmaceuticals for the money. The moment I got into pharmaceutical sales, I did what I could do in a very short time to prove who I was and what I could do. My mom spent her life in pharmaceutical sales, and I guess part of my path was choosing her path and showing her that I too could conquer what she had. By the time I got married and had my first baby, I was well on my way in my career to being CEO at the age of 30 which was my plan. By the time I went on my first mat leave, I was about to win an award and be the rockstar performer that I wanted to be. However, having my first baby changed my entire being from the inside out, and going back to work after 2 children in 3 years flipped my entire world upside down.

This is the moment where what society planned for me and what my authentic self needed were completely disconnected. I can only see it now looking back, that the mom I wanted to be and the mom that I'd become were so very different. To my 29-year-old self the word failure did not exist, I was always moving forward, pushing forward, driving forward on the path I had planned and the dreams I had envisioned for myself.

I think the best description is that I tried to be a superwoman in every aspect of my life and I failed miserably, but it was the best gift I would ever give myself.

I am sad that there's such separation in the world. Society tries to make us conform. The evolution of society, the pedestal…it's all fake, it's a lie. And what do these impossible standards teach us? To feel unworthy, to have body issues, to hate ourselves. It's not sustainable.

Authentic Self

All we want as human beings is to be our authentic selves. Society teaches us to squash ourselves and conform, from the time we're children to becoming adults. Then we need to strip it all away in order to find our true selves again.

Everyone has lived their life differently. Maybe you have conformed less. Maybe you have conformed more. There is no judgement here.

You have power. The power to become your authentic self again and watch everything that is meant for you come to you.

The gap between our authentic selves and what society tells us we must be is where we can find great opportunity. This is why so many of us get sick because the gap gets so big. The universe is screaming at us and our bodies are yelling. And my body was yelling very loudly...

HEART: Re-alignment

What do I dislike about my current work environment? Which tasks am I required to do that make me feel icky? What are the core beliefs behind the feeling? What do I love about my job? Where do I excel? Do the things I love outweigh the things I don't love? Am I at the right company but in the wrong role? Am I in the right role but the wrong company or industry? Am I in the right industry but the wrong company or role? Make some notes about your answers to these questions…

_____

_____

_____

_____

_____

_____

_____

_____

_____

_____

_____

Chapter 6: Human Emotions

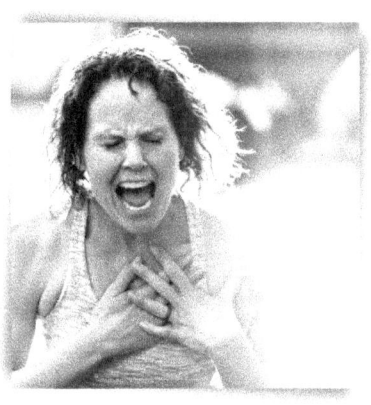

Photo Credit: Sophia MacAulay

Did you know there are 27 officially recognized emotions in this world that we have the pleasure of experiencing as human beings? Admiration, adoration, aesthetic appreciation, amusement, anger, anxiety, awe, awkwardness, boredom, calmness, confusion, craving, disgust, empathic pain, entrancement, excitement, fear, horror, interest, joy, nostalgia, relief, romance, sadness, satisfaction, sexual desire, and surprise,[7] as well as others that might fall in between or outside of these like grief, shame, jealousy, frustration, hopelessness, and hopefulness (to name a few).

I remember discovering this with my daughter at the psychologist's office and pretty much sinking in my chair. I believed, until then, that there were only 2—anger and happiness.

So many of us at my age were taught the same thing: if you were angry, go to your room; if you are happy, go out into the world. We were taught NOT to express, NOT to welcome the negative emotions, which means we ended up stuffing our emotions versus feeling them. It has become so subconscious for us that now we aren't even aware of the emotions we hold. This was NOT wrong, and this isn't our parents' fault. It was their own trauma and their own way that felt right at the time. And yet, for so many of us it's why we are stuck where we are.

---

[7] Anwar, Y. (2017, Sept. 6). Emoji fans take heart: Scientists pinpoint 27 states of emotion. *Berkeley News*. Retrieved from https://news.berkeley.edu/2017/09/06/27-emotions/

For a very long time, I held a lot of anger and wasn't even aware it was there. My kids certainly remember my moments of anger and we often talk about how blessed we are that I don't carry them anymore. There were days I'd slam doors and act like a 15-year-old kid. Other days, I'd walk in the door feeling happy and flip the switch within minutes because one small thing went wrong.

At the time, I had trouble seeing my anger. I knew I wasn't happy; however, I was numbing myself so much that I wasn't able to see that anger was overtaking most of my time at home with my family— who mattered most.

Brene Brown says, "We cannot selectively numb emotions; when we numb the painful emotions, we also numb the positive emotions."[8] I had trouble believing this as I thought I was actually feeling. I was actually doing interviews at the time at work for work/life balance because so many couldn't see how I was effectively getting my work done and not hanging on by a string and yet, I was doing it with NUMBNESS inside. Work wasn't seeing my

---

[8] Brown, B. (2010). *The Gifts of Imperfection*. Hazelden.

unhappiness because I showed up there with such excitement and drive, however, home was slowly withering away and I had no idea what to do so I chose to ignore it all...

I remember the day I consciously chose work over my family. I hate failing–I think we all do and yet, I was really struggling as a mom. Work was easy for me. It allowed me to be this person I felt proud of. Being a mom felt like endless failure and I disliked failure so I avoided it like the plague. The hardest thing as a mom is knowing you can't walk away. There were so many moments my kids and husband saw a side of me that I hid from the world and it was so much easier to run away instead of feeling the feelings...

You know by now that I wasn't blessed to start motherhood the way I had planned. I couldn't wait to have kids. I couldn't wait to be a mom and yet, on the day it happened, my entire life shifted. I ended up with PTSD in the delivery room. I remember how this felt and I remember the immediate numbness that came after this moment. After that, I went completely into automatic mode and couldn't feel

> anything. I flowed through having 2 beautiful daughters after that moment, moving as a family, starting a new job and trying to become the superhero of my life while barely holding on.
>
> I chose to NUMB it all.
>
> I wasn't taught how to feel and, looking back, it was the greatest lesson my soul ever chose to embrace.
>
>

Listen to Your Emotions

As kids, we weren't really taught how to emotionally regulate. It's not our parents' fault; they weren't taught it either.

I wasn't given the blessing of learning emotions and how to regulate until after the age of 36—sitting in my psychologist's office with my daughter because of course she didn't know how to regulate either.

I remember listening to what he was teaching and almost falling over in my chair when I realized I hadn't learned this valuable knowledge. It was life shifting...

Emotions are our body's way of communicating. When emotions arise, we are being asked to tune in, to discover what we need to pay attention to. If we choose to pay attention and feel the emotion we are being asked to feel, we can move forward empowered. If we block the emotion, over time they get built up inside, and eventually we no longer have space within.

Emotions that don't get dealt with become NUMBED, and ones that do teach us lessons to move forward and do it differently next time. We are meant to flow in our emotions, not HOLD them...

WOW.

Most of us right now are numbing and holding. We are either on pills to cope or using anger as our guiding force. I am not criticizing or judging in any way shape or form because I know that sometimes we need tools to move forward (remember at one point I was on 100mg of antidepressants too). However, I am asking that if you are numbing or full of anger—that NOW, you wake up and do something about it.

Remember, our kids are a mirror reflection of who we are...

What if the mirror our kids are reflecting can become our greatest gift in growing?
What if they are here to show us the good, bad, and ugly for us to see it and empower change in it.

Our kids are resilient, however they learn how to BE from watching us. If we are only using ANGER or NUMBNESS, they too will only choose ANGER or NUMBNESS.

We need to empower humans with the trauma that we hold and the opportunity in that trauma. So many of us walk around dead inside, so many of us walk around lost and don't know how to do this thing called life, and we don't talk about it so we sit on the couch and stare at the wall and wonder if this is normal.
What if nothing happens to you...what if it all happens for you? What is it going to take for you to learn and grow, to show up differently, for you to finally HEAL? This is our greatest opportunity...

Polarity

What if today, instead of feeling the shame around how you've shown up in the past, you did something about it?

What if you made a decision to dive a little deeper into the emotions you aren't feeling and wrapped your head around why? When we choose to grow, our kids automatically grow with us, as we are their guides and we all HEAL. For me, I have watched myself truly AGE backwards as I heal. I can tell you, it's very worth it.

On my healing journey, I have realized a powerful opportunity we have with the way we see our emotions. Emotions are perceptions of what is around us. If we choose to see something as "bad," then we often find ourselves stuck until the energy shifts. When we choose to see it differently, the energy shifts and so do the emotions. Wayne W. Dyer said, "When you change the way you look at things, the things you look at change." As I've grown and unravelled, I realized that the faster I choose to feel the emotion through a different lens—a lens of lessons or higher vibration emotions—I end up getting through the HARD much faster too. I end up being able to flow through it, accept it, make peace, and let it go differently.

Emotions have an opposite—a polarity—and the more you understand your emotions, the better you are able to choose the opposing emotion as a way to move through its partner:

1. Joy and sadness,
2. Acceptance and disgust,
3. Fear and anger,
4. Surprise and anticipation.[9]

Have you ever felt both excited and nervous? Lean into the excitement and don't focus so much on the nervousness. Focus instead on what the nervousness is trying to tell you.

If you are feeling angry, why? Is it really anger, or is it fear? Or deep profound sadness? The more you get to know your emotions, the easier it will be to talk about the real issues and flow through the emotion rather than letting it dictate how you show up.

---

[9] Karimova, H. (2017, Dec. 24). The Emotion Wheel: What It Is and How to Use It. *Positive Psychology*. Retrieved from https://positivepsychology.com/emotion-wheel/

I watched as I started to unlearn my anger and sadness and feel my way through it, so did my girls. As I shifted, they did too…as I learned, they did also.

It was magical to watch and that's why I unravelled it all…it started because of them and now I am most proud to feel it within me.

What if today, you took all the effort and people-pleasing ways you so easily give away to others and turned it back on yourself to start feeling again???

What if you stopped making yourself feel like a failure for the mistakes you've made and you faced your truths—the ones you are hiding from…

What if today, you allowed your emotions to flow and you used the HARD as the opportunity to listen, choosing to flow with the emotions where HIGHER vibrations are felt.
This is the choice we have…

HUMANS have polarity as well. We have a hard time accepting ourselves as both good and bad…we tend to get stuck in the emotions of failure or shame over things we've done. And yet learning how to accept that each one of us is the same is a great opportunity to shift out of the energy of misalignment. When we accept our polarity as humans, we truly accept and become our authentic selves. This is a daily practice since flowing with these emotions isn't easy and having the awareness to catch yourself will guide you to the person you are meant to be.

Let it Flow

This is what I had to do.

- I had to become selfish and allow the deep darkness to flow for the light to eventually shine through...
- I had to feel it all…
- Deal with it all…
- Accept my role in it all...
- Allow it all to flow…

This took 5 years, tonnes of counselling, meditation, mindfulness; you name it—I did it…however I DID IT!

You are worthy of the same...

As I unravelled the anger, the sadness, the depression, and the shame, I recognized a powerful force in being human that I was ignoring and maybe you are too.

We must feel to heal. We must feel to grow. We must feel in order to show up better for our children. When we grow, our children grow too.

We are HUMAN. Being human means that we are allowed to have these feelings that most of us ignore and yet, we can't live in them.

My mom always said powerful words that guided me through those moments when I wasn't acting as my mature self: "It's not what you do in the moment that matters most, it's what you do after that has the opportunity to shift it all."

What if today, the only thing you did differently is know you're not alone and move forward differently than the last time you felt the anger.
Today in my home, anger flows and no longer holds. It's the most incredible superpower we've developed within our home.

With my girls, we now talk a lot. We call each other out on our moments and, when we need guidance, we work through them together. We don't raise our voices. Instead, we use our words, articulate our emotions, and move forward together.

You are worthy of the same...

We can't change what has happened, however, we can empower what happens next.

Today, I empower you with the choice to do it differently and the opportunity to move forward. The time is now and our kids deserve it, now, more than ever...

So let the anger flow...
Feel the power of being HUMAN…
Know that you aren't alone...
Know that choice and perspective lie underneath it all…
Know that you are the only one who can empower it all…
The time is NOW…
You are so very worthy of it.

HEART: Human Experience

What emotions do you feel most often? What is the polarity of those? Does that surprise you? Write a statement that begins with: I feel _____ when I OR because of...

What about the emotions you don't often feel? When was the last time you remember feeling each of these and what prompted that feeling?

_____
_____
_____
_____
_____
_____
_____
_____
_____
_____